SALVAGE THAT FOOT

MISS STELLA ADAEZE IKE

1.0 INTRODUCTION

1.1 Salvaging the foot.

Deres Winston, being one of my patients was a Forty-three years old with a hole on his right foot. He started smoking and drinking when he was Nineteen years old. Had struggled with obesity for most of his life. At one point of his of mid-thirties, he was hounded by a company to recover #100, 000000 in debts. An old resume listed his longest job as lasting less than a year.

George M. Fifty eight years an architect, also my patient, presented with chronic ulcerated big toe in the hospital after a long time for dressing but in the process it was noticed that the entire foot was necrosed, blood supply has been cut off with lots of dead tissues. The whole process of necrosis was explained to Mr. George, the option was to do a thorough debridement, he left and did not come back until after two weeks.

Meanwhile, the infection spread to medial part of the right limb due to the uncontrolled Blood sugar. By the time he came back, the foot was already gangrenous. (a state of total loss of blood supply to the affected area causing death of the tissues and all organs connected.) This eventually led to below knee amputation of that right limb.

Mrs. North Gifts' a female fifty years old teacher presented with 1cm ulcer under her foot at the early stage in the hospital when she noticed it, the wound was assessed, wound dressing done and Mrs North adhered to the instructions her foot got healed though it took a lot of time and cost of money to ensure that the wound is managed adequately the limb was not amputated.

This book shows effective way and the role of nurses' as part of the team in the management of diabetic foot ulcer, modified method of wound care for diabetic foot ulcer and ways of preventing sore from occurring. As a Nurse practitioner with an experience over eleven years working in a hospital where chronic diabetic foot ulcers patients have stayed longer in the hospital, some that led to amputation of the lower Limb or Ray amputation of the big toe, three toes and high cost of managing the wound for both hospital and the patients. But with the current advancement in technology of managing patients and the role nurses take have reduced the length of stay in the hospital, amputation, and cost for the patients. The following chapters of the book are so captivating! Let's us all go find out what these is all about.

2.0 CHAPTER ONE

2.0.1 OVERVIEW OF DIABETES

Diabetes is a chronic metabolic disease characterised by elevated levels of blood glucose (or blood sugar), which leads over time to serious damage to the heart, blood vessels, eyes, kidneys, and nerves.

According to World Health Organization, about 422 million

people worldwide have diabetes, the majority living in low- and middle-income countries and 1.6 million deaths are directly attributed to diabetes each year. Both the number of cases and the prevalence of diabetes have been steadily increasing over the past few decades.

Diabetes occurs either when the pancreas does not produce enough insulin or when the body cannot effectively use the insulin it produces. Insulin is a hormone that regulates blood sugar. Hyperglycaemia, or raised blood sugar is a common effect of uncontrolled diabetes and over time leads to serious damages to many of the body's systems, especially the nerves and blood vessels.

In 2014, 8.5% of adult aged 18years and older had diabetes. In 2016, diabetes was the direct cause of 1.6 million deaths and in 2012 high blood glucose was the cause of other 2.2million deaths. Between 2000 and 2016, there was a 5% increase in premature mortality from diabetes in high-income countries the premature mortality rate due to diabetes decreased from 2000 to 2010 but then increased in 2010-2016. In lower-middle-income countries the premature mortality rate due to diabetes increased across from periods.

By contrast, the probability of dying from any one of the four main noncommunicable diabetes (cardiovascular diseases, cancer, chronic respiratory disease, or diabetes) between the ages of 30 and 70 decreased by 18% globally between 2000 and 2016. (Sarwar N, Gao P, Seshasai SR, et al 2010). The types of diabetes include: **TYPE 1 Diabetes**: This characterized by deficient insulin production and requires daily administration of insulin. Neither the cause of Type 1 diabetes nor the symptoms include excessive excretion of urine (polyuria), thirst (polydipsia), constant hunger, weight loss, vision changes and fatigue. These symptoms may occur suddenly. **TYPE 2 Diabetes**: This results from the body's ineffective use of insulin. Most people with diabetes is largely the result of excess body weight and physical inactivity. The symptoms in Type 2 may be like those of Type 1 diabetes but are often less marked. As a result, the disease may be diagnosed several years after onset, after complication has already arisen. Recently, this type of diabetes was seen only in adults, but it is now also occurring increasing frequently i children. **Gestational Diabetes**: This is hyperglycaemia with blood glucose values above normal but below those diagnostics of diabetes. Gestational diabetes occurs during pregnancy. Women with gestational diabetes are at increased risk of complications during pregnancy and at delivery. These women and possibly their children are also at increased risk of Type 2 diabetes in future. Gestational diabetes is diagnosed through prenatal screening, rather than through reported symptoms.

Impaired Glucose Tolerance and Impaired Fasting Glycaemia: Impaired glucose   tolerance (IGT) and impaired fasting glycaemia (IFG) are intermediate conditions in the transition between normality and diabetes. People with IGT or IFG are at high risk of progressing to Type 2 diabetes, although this is not inevitable

3.0 CHAPTER TWO

3.0.1 HOW DIABETIC FOOT ULCER DEVELOPS

A diabetic foot ulcer is an open sore or wound that occurs in approximately 15 percent of patients with diabetes and is commonly located on the bottom of the foot, toes. Diabetic foot disease is one of the most significant and devastating complications of diabetes. It is defined as a foot affected by ulceration that is associated with neuropathy and or peripheral arterial disease of the lower limb in a patient with diabetes. The term diabetic foot disease also refers to a mix of pathologies including diabetic neuropathy, peripheral vascular disease, foot ulceration, osteomyelitis, endpoint limb amputation and potentially preventable. The images below show diabetic foot ulcer process:

Figure 1

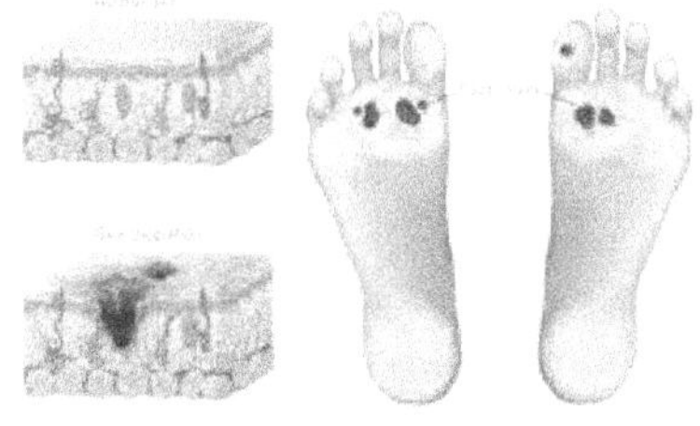

Figure 2
Shows how puerperal Neuropathy develops

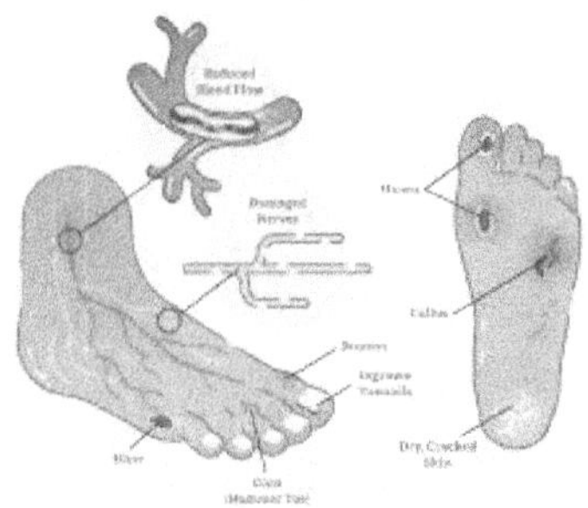

Diabetic foot problem in patients have remained a major public health issue and are most common reason for admission of diabetic patients in a hospital. The prevalence of diabetic foot ulceration in the diabetic population is 4-10%, with the peak prevalence being between 0 and 80 years of age. It is estimated that about 5% of all patients with diabetes present with a history of foot ulceration while the lifetime risk of diabetic patients developing this complication is 15%.

Most diabetic foot ulcers (60-80%) will heal while 10-155 of them will remain active and 5-24% of them will finally lead to amputation within the period of 6-18 months after first evaluation. Diabetes accounts for up to 80% non-traumatic amputation, with 85% of these being preceded
by a foot ulcer. Amputation carries with a significant elevated mortality at follow-up ranging from 13 to 40% at 1 year to 39.80% at 5 year

Figure 3

Necrosis diabetic foot of the left big toe

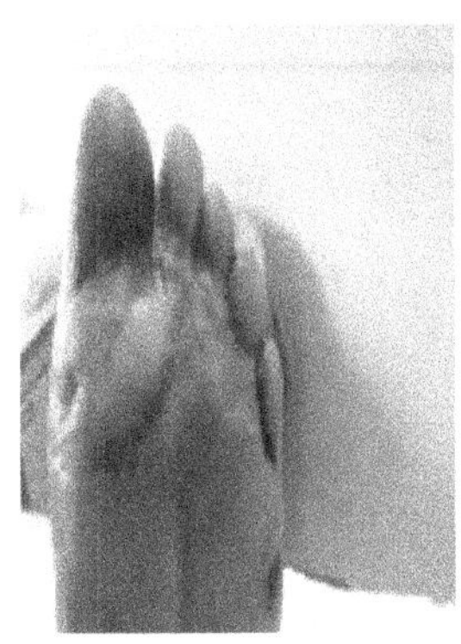

Figure 4

Diabetic Foot Ulcer

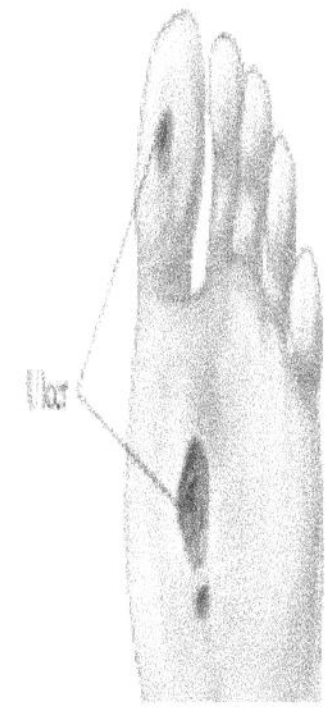

Figure 5

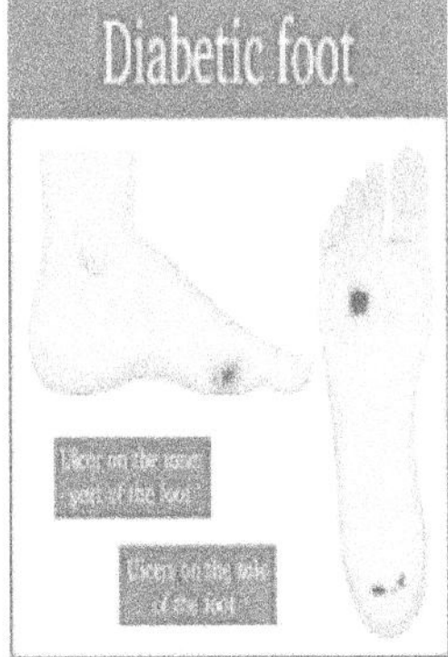

Figure 6 stages of diabetic foot ulcer

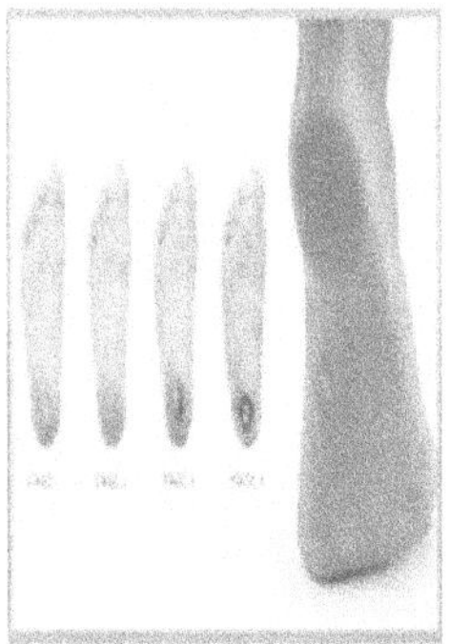

Figure 7 shows the spread of infection and Ray amputation of the big toe

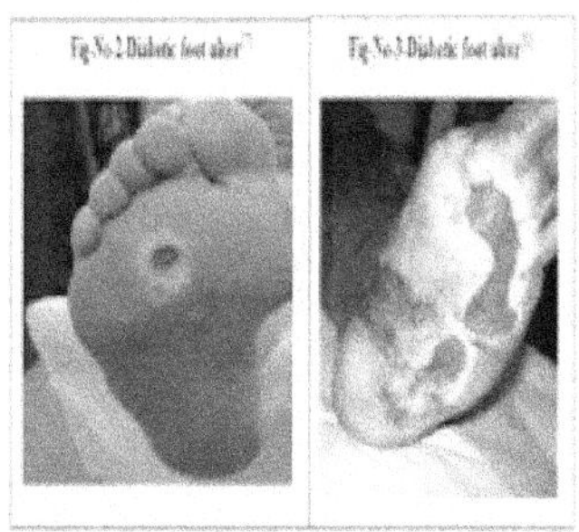

Figure 8

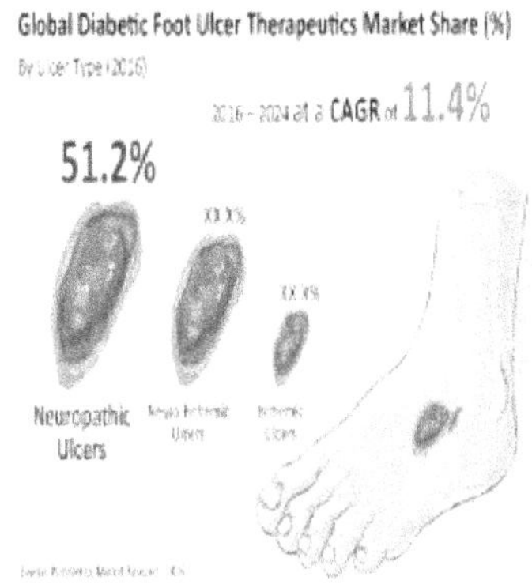

Figure 9

indicates the angiopathic pathway of diabetic foot ulcer

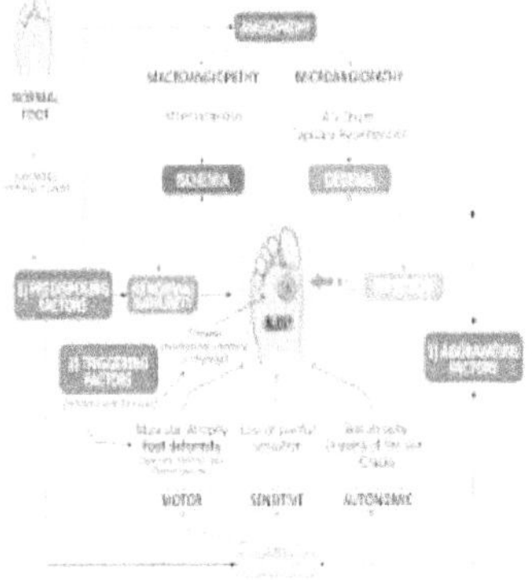

3.1 CAUSES OF DIABETIC FOOT ULCER

- Lack feeling in the foot (Peripheral Neuropathy)
- Poor circulation (Peripheral vascular system)
- High blood sugar (Hyperglycaemia)
- Trauma
- Irritation (friction and pressure)

3.1.2 RISK FACTORS FOR DIABETIC FOOT   ULCERS

- Poorly fitted or poor-quality shoes
- Poor hygiene (not washing regularly or thoroughly)
- Improper trimming of toenails
- Alcohol consumption
- Eye disease from diabetes

- Heart disease
- Kidney disease
- Obesity
- Tobacco use (inhibits blood circulation)
- Common in older men

3.1.3 The tables below show different risk factors and predominant site for ulceration

Table 1 shows the differences in risk factors for diabetic foot ulcer

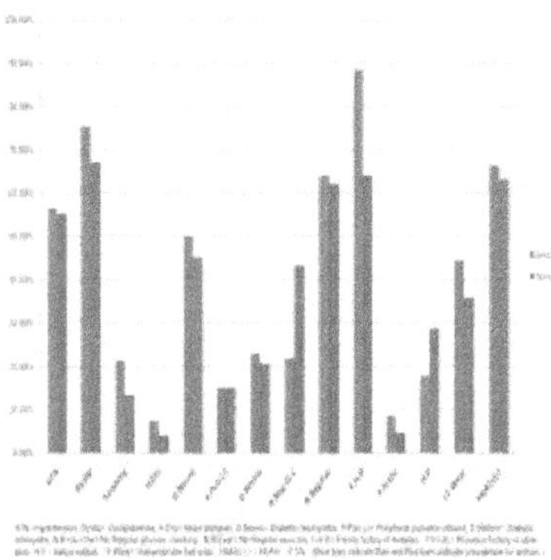

Table 2

The predominant site for ulcer localization was the dorsum (n=36; 34.6%) followed by sole of foot (n=24; 23.1%

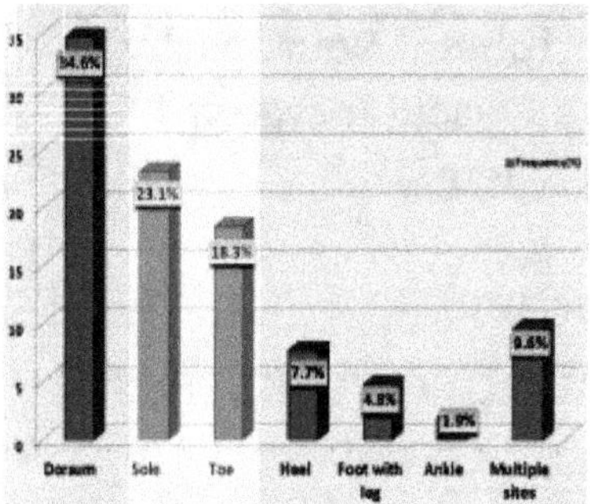

3.1.4 CLASSIFICATIONS OF DIABETIC FOOT ULCER
There are two most established classification systems they are:
  a. The Meggitt-Wagner
  b. University of Texas systems

3.1.5 ADVANCED CLASSIFICATION OF DIABETIC FOOT ULCER

    c. Diabetic Ulcer Severity Score Classification
    d. Site Ischemia, Neuropathy, Bacterial Infection and Depth Wound Classification

3.1.6 WAGNER-MEGGITT CLASSIFICATION

It was developed in the 1970s, been the most widely accepted and grading systems for lesions of the diabetic foot. The first four grades (grade 0, 1. 2, and 3) are based on the physical depth of the lesion in and through soft tissues of the foot. The last two grades (grade 4 and 5) are completely distinct because they are based on the extent of gangrene and lost perfusion in the foot. Grade 4 refers to partial and Grade 5 refers to a completely gangrenous foot. The gap in Wagner-Meggitt classification is that it did not address all diabetic foot ulcerations and infections. The tabular classification of diabetic foot ulcer

Grade 0	Intact skin
Grade 1	Superficial ulcers
Grade 2	Deep ulcers
Grade 3	Ulcer with bone involvement
Grade 4	Forefoot gangrene
Grade 5	Full foot gangrene

3.1.7 UNIVERSITY OF TEXAS SYSTEM CLASSIFICATION

The University of Texas Classifications represents an advance in the treatment of diabetic foot. This system uses four grades, each of which is modified by the presence of, infection (Stage B), ischemia (Stage C) or both (Stage D)- Since the increasing grade and stage of wounds are less likely to heal without revascularization or amputation,

Stage	Grade			
	0	I	II	III
A	Pre- or post-ulcerative lesion completely epithelialized	Superficial wound not involving tendon, capsule or bone	Wound penetrating to tendon or capsule	Wound penetrating to bone or joint
B	Infection	Infection	Infection	Infection
C	Ischemia	Ischemia	Ischemia	Ischemia
D	Infection and ischemia	Infection and ischemia	Infection and ischemia	Infection and ischemia

3.1.8 **DIABETIC ULCER SEVERITY SCORE CLASSIFICATION**

The Diabetic Ulcer Severity Score (DUSS) is based on the categorization of wounds into specific severity subgroups for a comparison of outcomes. Assessment using the (DUSS9) systems includes the presence of pedal pulse, the ability to probe to bone within the ulcer, and ulcer quantity and location. The sum of point determines severity, with the score ranging from 0-4

Parameter	Score=0	Score =1
Palpable pedal pulse	Present	Absent
Probing to bone	No	Yes
Ulcer site	Toes	Foot
Ulcer number	Single	Multiple

3.1.9 **SITE ISCHEMIA, NEUROPATHY, BACTERIA INFECTION AND DEPTH WOUND CLASSIFICATION**

The site, ischemia, neuropathy, bacterial infection uses five clinical features which are graded as either present or(0) or absent (1) The maximum score is 6 A representative of classification is as follows:

Clinical Features	Score=0	Score=1
Site	Forefoot	Midfoot or hindfoot
Ischemia	Pedal blood flow intact; at least one pulse palpable	Clinical evidence of reduced pedal blood flow
Neuropathy	Protective sensation intact	Protective sensation lost
Bacterial infection	None	Present
Area	Less than 1cm2	Greater than 1cm2
Depth	Skin and subcutaneous	Reaching muscle, tendon, or deeper

4.0 CHAPTER THREE

4.1 ROLE OF NURSES' IN WOUND CARE/ DRESSSING OF DIABETIC FOOT ULCER

The science of wound care has advanced significantly over the past ten years. The old thought of " let the air get at it" is now known to be harmful. We know that wounds and ulcers heal faster, with a lower risk of infection. The use of full-strength betadine, hydrogen peroxide, whirlpools and soaking are not recommended, as these practices could lead to further complications.

Improvement of patient care and health services are one of the most important aspect of Nursing. According to World Health Organization, nurses are the largest groups in the in the world who are involved in different levels of health. Obviously, there are several reasons for the presence of nurses in the health care team. Generally, the four major goals are including health promotion, prevention of diseases, patients care and simply patients' compliance. There are seven main roles for nurses include 1. Providing health care, 2. Care connector, 3. Educator, 4. Consultant, 5. Leader, 6. Researcher, 7. Supporting the rights of patient. So, nurses play important role to manage diabetes and diabetes nursing is divided into several categories, including nurse practitioner, clinical nurse specialist, diabetic nurse, generalist nurse, and each has clear duties. Nurses are actively involved in the prevention and early detection of diabetes and its complication. Nurses play their educating role in the field of prevention of diabetic foot, foot care and preventing from foot injury, early detection of any changes in skin and foot sensation, dressing, help patient sufferings from diabetic foot ulcer or amputation,

4.1.2 Nurse's Role in Education

Nurses have an effective role in prevention of foot ulcers and lower limb amputation by educational intervention, screening high-risk people and providing health care. There is no doubt that diabetes education is an essential aspect of diabetes management. One of the goals of Healthy People 2020 is to increase the proportion of diabetes patients receiving formal diabetes education from 56.8% to 62.5%. The importance of foot care education is stressed by the International Diabetes Federation. Nurse encourages self-management education as extremely important because patient and their relatives provide a high percentage of caregiving. The team inclusive of nurses in the management of diabetic foot ulcer needs thorough education and training as the play a key role. The main goal of it is to increase staff awareness of the diabetic foot ulcer risks and improve their skills in examination and treatment of diabetic foot ulcer. One of the aims of education is to change behaviour and promote self-management because it was reported that poor foot care is associated with high-risk ulcerations, amputations, and mortality.

4.1.3 Nurse's Role in Examination and Screening

Peripheral neuropathy, peripheral vascular disease and infection are three major factors for diabetic foot ulcer that can lead to gangrene and amputation. However, peripheral neuropathy is solely responsible for more than 80% of foot ulcer in diabetic ulcer. It is not only important for neurological examination as the first criterion for screening patients at risk for foot ulcers. But on the emphasis on nurse's role in performing a diabetic foot examination monofilament and collaboration with other diabetic foot ulcer members. Diabetic foot examination should be part of all visits. Nurses should ask patient to remove their shoes and socks and then examine their feet to screen patients at high risk and report to other member of the multidisciplinary diabetic foot team.

4.1.4 Nurses Cooperation In Diabetic Foot Treatment

Nurse produces an excellent diabetic foot care to be the complimentary care

Wound dressing represents a part of the management of diabetic foot ulceration. In choosing dressings, several factors ought to be considered according to the type of ulcers have to be considered. An infected wound tends to have heavy exudates that need to be controlled to prevent maceration of the surrounding tissue. There may be considerable odour associated with infection. However, proper management of infected diabetic foot ulcers should include appropriate antibiotic therapy, regular and thorough debridement, and daily wound dressing changes. It is imperative to evaluate the arterial and venous status of the affected limb. This will help determine the appropriate medical and potential surgical treatment. Desirable characteristics for wound dressings must incorporate the principle of wound healing. Dressings have since been engineered to maintain the moist environment while also controlling the growth of microorganism, allowing gaseous exchange, and thermally insulating the wound, which allows atraumatic removal.

4.1.5 Nurses' Role in Rehabilitation

The role of the nurse is to in helping patient with diabetic foot ulcer is to have movement. This vital especially for patients, who have lost their foot, Nurses should identify different types of devices and its applications to introduce to the patients based on patient conditions to maintain their mobility. Nurses encourage and teach the patient the use of assistive devices. As a diabetic foot nurse, their duties in the field includes: the introduction, training, and participation of patients in the make, use of devices such as cane, walkers and wheelchair (which completely remove pressure on the limb) along with the aids such as shoes, boots, the Scottish stone, and full contact plaster.

5.0 DEBRIDEMENT

Debridement is the removal of necrotic tissue, foreign debris, bacterial growth, callus, wound edge, and wound bed tissue from chronic wounds to stimulate the wound healing process. Stimulation of wound healing mediated by debridement is thought to occur by the conversion of a chronic non-healing wound environment to an acute healing environment through the removal of cells that are not responsive to endogenous healing stimuli. Debridement is used commonly in standard wound treatment of diabetic foot ulcers (DFUs).

It can also be a surgical management as indicated for debridement of nonviable and infected tissue from the ulceration, removal of excess callus, curettage of underlying osteomyelitis bone, skin grafting, and revascularization. The wound usually requires an initial surgical debridement and probing to determine the depth and involvement of bone or joint structures. Visible or palpable bone implies an 85% chance of osteomyelitis.

5.1 METHODS OF DEBRIDEMENT

- Surgery (sharp debridement)
- Chemical debridement (antiseptics, polysaccharide beads, pastes)
- Autolytic (hydrogels, hydrocolloids, and trans-

parent films),
- Biosurgery (maggots)
- Mechanical (hydro debridement),
- Biochemical debridement (enzyme preparations)
- Enzymatic debridement: Collagen comprises a significant fraction of the necrotic soft tissues in chronic wounds; the enzyme collagenase, derived from fermentation of *Clostridium histolyticum*, helps remove nonviable tissue from the surface of wounds. However, it is not a substitute for an initial surgical excision of a grossly necrotic wound.

Callus is a build-up of keratinized skin formed under conditions of repeated pressure or friction and may contribute to ulcer formation by creating focal areas of high plantar pressure. The debridement of callus has been proposed to be relevant for both treatment and prevention of DFU. After debridement, apply a moist sodium chloride dressing or isotonic sodium chloride gel (example, Norm gel, IntraSite gel) or a hydro active paste (example, Duoderm). Optimal wound coverage requires wet-to-damp dressings, which support autolytic debridement, absorb exudate, and protect surrounding healthy skin. A polyvinyl film dressing (example, OpSite, Tegaderm) that is semi permeable to oxygen and moisture and impermeable to bacteria is a good choice for wounds that are neither very dry nor highly exudative. Wound coverage recommendations for some other wound conditions.

5.1.2 PRESSURE OFFLOADING IN DIABETIC FOOT ULCER

- For patients with a neuropathic plantar ulcer, a non-removable knee-high offloading device—i.e., either a total contact cast (TCC) or a removable walker that is rendered irremovable by the provider who fits the device is the preferred offloading treatment

- In patients who cannot tolerate a non-removable, knee-high offloading device, or if such a device is contraindicated, a removable version can be considered; should a removable device be contraindicated or if it cannot be tolerated, an ankle-high offloading device can be considered; patients must be educated with regard to the benefits of adherence to removable device use
- While offloading remains important in the presence of infection or ischemia, greater caution is necessary
- Non plantar foot ulcers, depending on their type and location, should be addressed with a removable, ankle-high offloading device, footwear modifications, toe spacers, or orthoses
- When ankle pressure is below 50 mmHg or the ankle brachial index (ABI) is less than 0.5, urgent vascular imaging and, in the presence of appropriate findings, revascularization, should be considered; revascularization should also be considered if the toe pressure is below 30 mmHg or the transcutaneous pressure of oxygen (TcpO$_2$) is less than 25 mmHg; however, revascularization may be considered at higher pressures should extensive tissue loss or infection occur
- If optimal treatment does not result in ulcerative healing signs within 6 weeks, revascularization should be considered, regardless of the outcomes of the above-mentioned vascular tests
- If an above-the-ankle amputation is being contemplated, revascularization should first be considered as an option
- Revascularization should be avoided in patients with an unfavourable risk-benefit ratio
- Individual factors (example, morphologic distribution of peripheral artery disease, autogenous vein availability, patient comorbidities) and local operator expertise

should be considered when selecting a revascularization technique

- Following revascularization, perfusion should be objectively measured to assess the procedure's effectiveness
- Smoking cessation, hypertension and dyslipidaemia control, and antiplatelet drug use, as the means to reduce cardiovascular risk, should be emphasized
- For a superficial ulcer with limited soft tissue (mild) infection - The ulcer should be cleansed and all necrotic tissue and surrounding callus should be debrided; start empiric oral antibiotic therapy directed against *Staphylococcus aureus* and streptococci (unless there are indications that alternative or additional likely pathogens exist)
- For deep or extensive (potentially limb-threatening) infection (moderate or severe infection) - The need for surgical intervention to remove necrotic tissue, including infected bone, should be urgently evaluated, and compartment pressure should be released or abscesses drained; assess for peripheral artery disease (with urgent treatment, including revascularization, to be considered if such disease is present); empiric, parenteral, broad-spectrum antibiotic therapy aimed at common gram-positive and gram-negative bacteria, including obligate anaerobes, should be initiated; the clinical response to empirical therapy, along with culture and sensitivity results, should be used to adjust (constrain and target, if possible) the antibiotic regimen with regard to local ulcer care.
- The ulcer must be inspected regularly by a trained health-care provider, with the severity of the ulcer, the underlying pathology, the presence of infection, the amount of exudation, and wound treatment provided determining the frequency of examination
- Ulcer debridement and removal of the surrounding callus (preferably with sharp surgical instruments) should be carried out, with the procedure repeated as necessary

- Selected dressings should control excess exudation and keep the environment moist
- Negative pressure should be considered as an aid to healing postoperative wounds
- If noninfected ulcers do not heal after 4-6 weeks of optimal clinical care, one of the following adjunctive treatments should be considered - If severe ischemia is not present in a neuro-ischemic ulcer, a sucrose octasulfate–impregnated dressing; if moderate ischemia is either present or absent, a multi-layered patch of autologous leucocytes, platelets, and fibrin; also in the presence of absence of moderate ischemia, placental membrane allografts; in ischemic ulcers in which revascularization has not led to healing, adjunctive treatment with systemic oxygen therapy

6.1 Management of Systemic and Local Factors

Treatment of diabetic foot ulcers requires management of several systemic and local factors.

Precise diabetic control is, of course, vital, not only in achieving resolution of the current wound, but also in minimizing the risk of recurrence. Management of contributing systemic factors, such as hypertension, hyperlipidaemia, atherosclerotic heart disease, obesity, or renal insufficiency, is crucial. Management of arterial insufficiency, treatment of infection with appropriate antibiotics, offloading the area of the ulcer, and wound care are also essential.

Options for Soft Tissue Coverage of the Clean but Nonhealing Wound

Once a wound has reached a steady clean state, a decision must be made about allowing healing by natural processes or expediting healing by a surgical procedure. Clinical experience and observation of the healing progress in each case dictate the appropriate management. Surgical options include skin grafting, application of bioengineered skin substitutes, and flap closures.

Skin grafts

5.2 TYPES OF DRESSING FOR DIABETIC FOOT ULCERATIONS

6.3 Nonadherent or Low-adherence Dressing

Nonadherent or saline soaked gauze are often regarded as standard treatment for diabetic ulcers and designed to be atraumatic. These simple, relatively inexpensive dressings are not designed specifically for managing infection can be used in conjunction with antibiotic treatments. Non adherent dressings are basically a low adherent wound pad for pain-free removal of the dressing, and it is mostly used for minor wounds. These dressings have been designed to protect the fragile tissue in wounds therefore minimising trauma upon removal of the dressing or the need for dressing changes. They are designed for draining or scabbed wounds and are highly absorbent to keep the wound dry. The dressing will not disrupt the healing tissue by sticking to the wound and they are also ideal as a primary dressing for lightly draining wounds.

Sterile non-adherent dressings are ideal for use on both first- and second-degree burns. It protects the fragile tissue in wounds with its unique structure. It has an advanced mesh design which is extremely comfortable for the patient and which minimises the risk of any exudates (fluid leaking from a wound) pool and the secondary dressing having adherence to the wound. It is associated with patient comfort and minimal pain at dressing removal.

Non adherent dressings can also be utilised in the management of traumatic wounds, including skin tears and in patients with fragile or friable skin. Any adherence of the dressing material to the skin can disrupt the formation of new cells leading to stripping of the epidermal layer and causing distress to the patient. These dressings are gentle on the skin and are suitable for use in patients with a high risk of sensitivity, such as those with leg ulcers thus minimising tissue maceration.

5.2.1 Hydrocolloid Dressing

Hydrocolloid dressing is semi permeable to vapour, occlusive to wound exudates and absorbent, they are usually presented as an absorbent layer on a form. They were found to be second most popular choice of dressing. Despite their popularity, their use on infected wounds is controversial,

Hydrocolloid materials are designed to be occlusive, trapping exudates within the dressing and hydrating the wound. This creates a hypoxic and moist environment that may also facilitate autolysis of necrotic materials. However, concern that hydrocolloids may increase the risk of infection developing within a wound. Not recommended for wounds with heavy exudates, sinus tracts must be used with caution on the feet of patients with diabetes. It's suggested that hydrocolloid dressings can be used safely on diabetic foot ulcers if 1. they are used only on appropriate wounds after a thorough patient assessment, 2. the wound is superficial with no signs of infection, 3. there is low to moderate exudates, 4. there are no signs or symptoms of ischemia and 5. dressings are done frequently.

5.2.2 How to apply a hydrocolloid dressing

Wash your hands and put on gloves.
Remove the soiled dressing (noting the date it was applied) and place it in a trash bag.
Remove your gloves, wash your hands, and put on new gloves.
Clean the wound with normal saline
solution or prescribed cleanser.
Use clean gauze to pat dry the tissue surrounding the wound.
Remove your gloves, wash your hands, and put on new gloves.
Apply liquid barrier film or moisture barrier to the peri wound area.
For deep wounds, apply wound filler or packing materials as indicated.

Before applying the hydrocolloid dressing, warm it by holding it between your hands to increase adhesive ability.
Remove the paper backing from the dressing.
Gently fold the dressing in half lengthwise and apply it from the centre of the wound outward.
Smooth the dressing in place from the centre outward. Hold the dressing in place for a few seconds to improve
adhesion.
The dressing should be at least 1 inch larger than the wound. (Some manufacturers may require a 2-inch border.)
You may apply tape around the edges to secure the dressing.
Dispose of the waste.
Remove your gloves and discard.

5.2.3 Hydrogels Dressing

They are like hydrocolloid dressing in that they are designed to facilitate autolysis of necrotic tissue, but the differ in that the donate moisture to extensively dry wounds. Examples Aqua form (Maersk Medical) and Intrasite Gel (Smith and Nephew). Thus, they can lead to maceration when applied to wounds that are moderately to heavily exudating. Their use on a diabetic foot lesion should be an adjunct to sharp debridement of necrotic eschar. The benefits of using hydrogel-based dressings for wound care are vast, especially if you know how to administer the gel properly. An excellent source for providing moisture to a dry lesion, hydrogel dressings act fast to help cool down a wound, as well as provide temporary relief from pain for up to six hours. Here are a few quick guidelines on when to use hydrogel dressings, its wound healing advantages and when you should try to abstain from using hydrogel.

Hydrogel dressings consist of 90 percent water in a gel base, according to the medical journal Apple Bites, and serves to help monitor fluid exchange from within the wound surface. By keeping the wound moist, the hydrogel dressing assists in protecting your body from wound infection and promotes efficient healing.

Hydrogel dressings generally come in three different forms, including:

- Amorphous hydrogel: a free-flowing gel, distributed in tubes, foil packets and spray bottles
- Impregnated hydrogel: typically saturated onto a gauze pad, nonwoven sponge ropes and/or strips
- Sheet hydrogel: a combination of gel held together by a thin fibre mesh

Healing benefits

Because of the moisture provided to the wound from the hydrogel dressing, common healing phases such as granulation, epidermis repair and the removal of excess dead tissue become simplified. In addition to aiding the wound treatment stages, the cool sensation provided by the hydrogel to the wound offers relief from pain for at least six hours. When hydration is provided for the wound bed, discomfort experienced from changing the dressing becomes reduced, and the risk of infection also becomes decreased.

When to use

The following types of wounds are the most suited for being treated with hydrogel dressings:

➢ dry or dehydrated wounds
➢ partial or full-thickness lesions
➢ abrasions or severe scrapes
➢ minor burns
➢ wounds with granulated tissue development
➢ radiation skin damage

It is important to remember to avoid hydrogen dressing use when a wound is extremely moist or displaying heavy exudates. In most cases, hydrogel dressings will need a cover dressing because they are often difficult to secure and can dehydrate easily if not covered effectively.

Dressing changes

It is advised to change your hydrogel dressing no less often than every four days to stop the covering from becoming too close or attached to the injury site. You can essentially tell if it is time for a dressing change due to an abundance of fluid that indicates that the wound could be receiving too much hydration. If you are using an amorphous type hydrogel dressing, remember to rinse off any leftover gel with a wound cleanser or normal saline solution if necessary. As for removing the impregnated gauze or sheet hydrogel, gently lift an edge up and peel back slowly after soaking the covering in saline solution to help soften the bandage. Always remember to use general aseptic technique precautions when removing the dressing, such as washing your hands, wearing gloves, and disposing of the bandage immediately after taking it off.

5.2.4 Alginates Dressing

They are highly absorbent, pack into cavity wounds, provide haemostasis and are atraumatic at dressing change (but require wetting) Examples include Kaltostat (Convatec) and Sorbsan (Maersk Medical). It is important to ensure that all dressing is removed from a cavity wound, because retained dressing may be a source for further infection. Alginates dressing are absorbent wound care products that contain sodium and calcium fibres derived from seaweed. They come in the form of flat dressings that can be placed over open ulcers and rope dressings that are used for packing the wound, which absorb fluids and promote healing with pressure ulcers, diabetic foot ulcers, or venous ulcers. An individual dressing can absorb up to 20 times its own weight. These dressings, which are easy to use, mould themselves to the shape of the wound, which helps ensure that they absorb wound drainage properly. This also makes these dressings ideal for using on ulcers in areas that are difficult to dress, such as heels and sacral areas.

How Do Alginate Dressings Work?

Alginate dressings are dry when initially placed on an open wound and become larger and more gel-like as they draw in fluids. This helps clear out the wound, prevents it from becoming dry, and protects it from harmful bacteria, which helps lower the risk of infection. These dressings also help promote new skin growth during the wound healing process by ensuring that the wound area stays moist. This encourages natural debridement via enzymes, which supplements the wound care provided by wound care practitioners in a clinical setting. The debridement process removes dead or damaged skin, promoting a healthier wound environment that aids wound healing.

Alginate dressings can also help wounds that are bleeding. The calcium in these dressings helps stabilize blood flow, which slows bleeding.

How to Use an Alginate Dressing

- Treating wounds with alginate dressings is a straightforward process if you follow the correct wound care procedure using these steps:
- Use normal saline solution to clean the wound area.
- Pat the area around the wound dry.
- Place the alginate dressing over the wound.
- Secure a secondary dressing over the alginate dressing to hold it in place.
- Change the dressing everyone to three days, or when fluid starts to seep out from the edges of the dressings.
- Before removing the alginate during a dressing change, use saline to dampen it to lower the risk of damaging the surrounding skin.

Tips for Using Alginate Dressings

Keep in mind that alginate dressings are designed for use on draining wounds or wounds with excessive amounts of fluid. They should not be used on wounds that have very little drainage or they may dry them out, which slows the healing process. Although alginate dressings typically keep wounds moist for faster healing, they need to form a gel to do so. In some cases, this gel does not form, which increases the risk of having the dressing stick to the skin and cause irritation or damage.

6.0 MODIFIED WOUND CARE/ DRESSING DIABETIC FOOT ULCER MANAGEMENT

The management of diabetic foot ulcers requires offloading the wound by using appropriate therapeutic footwear, daily saline dressing to provide a moist wound environment, debridement when necessary, antibiotic therapy of osteomylities or cellulitis is present, optimal control of blood glucose and evaluation and correction of peripheral arterial insufficiency, Additionally, it causes less discomfort with moist wound dressing. **A** multidisciplinary (Endocrinologist, Podiatrist, Nurse, Vascular Surgeon, Microbiologist, Orthotist, Nutritionist) approach should be employed because of the multifaceted nature of the foot ulcer and the numerous co-morbidities that can occur in the patient.

ADVANCED THERAPIES FOR DIABETIC FOOT ULCERS

Vascular reconstruction

In general, the indications for vascular surgery in the presence of a constructible arterial lesion include intractable pain at rest or at night, intractable foot ulcers, and impending or existing gangrene. Intermittent claudication alone is only infrequently disabling and intractable enough to warrant bypass surgery. Physicians must specifically ask for symptoms suggestive of intermittent claudication, such as pain in the buttocks and thighs while walking and abatement of pain when at rest.

6.0 The autologous skin graft is the criterion standard for viable coverage of the partial thickness wound. The graft can be harvested under local anaesthesia as an outpatient procedure. Meshing the graft allows wider coverage and promotes drainage of serum and blood.

7.0 A cadaveric skin allograft is a useful covering for relatively deep wounds following surgical excision when the wound bed does not appear appropriate for application of an autologous skin graft. The allograft is, of course, only a temporary solution.

6.0 Wound coverage by cultured human cells.
Revisional Surgery

Revisional surgery for bony architecture may be required to remove pressure points. Such intervention includes resection of metatarsal heads or ostectomy

6.1 Hydrotherapy

Intractable, infected, cavity wounds sometimes improve with hydrotherapy using saline pulse lavage under pressure (PulsEvac).

6.1.2 Extracorporeal shock-wave therapy

Two multicentre, randomized, sham-controlled, double-blinded, phase III clinical trials by Snyder et al indicated that extracorporeal shock-wave therapy (ESWT) can effectively treat neuropathic diabetic foot ulcers that fail to heal with standard therapy alone. At 24 weeks, in patients with diabetic foot ulcers that had not been reduced by 50% or greater over the course of 2 weeks' standard treatment, complete healing occurred in 37.8% of patients treated with ESWT and standard care, compared with 26.2% of patients treated with sham therapy and standard care.

6.1.3 Cellular and/or Tissue-Based Products: Cellular and acellular-based, placental/amniotic/chorionic derived products decreases risk of amputation and increased wound closure when compared with generalized wound care standard

6.1.4 Collagen Product: Collagen dressing technology comes in different particles, pads, gels and gels support, it creates a scaffolding matrix that regulates extracellular components, therefore moving chronic wounds towards closure.

6.1.5 GROWTH FACTOR: Recombinant human platelet-derived growth factor-BB (rhPDGF-BB) (becaplermin) or Heterogenic dressing/graft, application of recombinant growth factors have been shown to lower chronic wounds. Becaplermin gel increase both complete wound closure and decrease the time to achieve complete.

6.1.6 Hyper oxygen therapy (HBOT) if arterial insufficiency is present. Benefit of this approach include prevention of tissue dehydration and cell death, acceleration of angiogenesis and facilitation of the growth factors with the target cells which has been proven to reduce amputation rates in patients with ischemic diabetic foot. It reduces wound Infection, Wound breakdown, Flip/Skin Graft loss, and Tissue Expand/Implant loss. It is done 30-60 sessions for optimal result in difficult wound

6.1.7 Negative Pressure Wound Therapy and Hyperbaric Oxygen

The use of negative pressure wound therapy devices may be useful in the treatment of non-healing wounds as they may reduce oedema, remove bacterial product, and draw the edges of wound together to promote closure. This method is considered when other treatments are not effective. Elective surgery to correct structural deformities that can be performed as needed in certain patients such as hammertoe repair, metatarsal osteotomies, planter exosteotomies and Achilles tendon lengthening

8.0 CHAPTER FOUR

8.1 Prevention

The best way to treat a diabetic foot ulcer is to prevent its development that leads to amputation. The best approach is through diabetic counselling which include:

- To make use of a team of multidisciplinary professionals who are committed to limb salvage
- Recommend guidelines include seeing a podiatrist
- Reducing: smoking drinking alcohol, high cholesterol, and elevated blood sugar
- Wearing of appropriate shoes to OFFLOAD PRESSURE and socks
- Learning how to check foot including debridement is crucial so to find potential problem as early as possible.
- Inspect the feet especially the soles and between the toes for (cuts, bruises, cracks, blisters, redness, ulcers, and any sign of abnormality).
- Regular visit to podiatrist
- Achieve and maintain healthy body weight

. Treatment of diabetic foot ulcers requires management of several systemic and local factors.

Precise diabetic control is, of course, vital, not only in achieving resolution of the current wound, but also in minimizing the risk of recurrence. Management of contributing systemic factors, such as hypertension, hyperlipidemia, atherosclerotic heart disease, obesity, or renal insufficiency, is crucial. Management of arterial insufficiency, treatment of infection with appropriate antibiotics, offloading the area of the ulcer, and wound.

9.0 CONCLUSION

Diabetic foot ulcer as the most common cause of hospitalization in diabetic patients that is one of the health systems concerns. The diabetic foot ulcer can be a burden, complex and expensive for both the patient and the clinician. If diabetic foot ulcers are not prevented, identified early, professionally managed and treated as appropriate, complications can lead to infection, amputation, and even death. Advanced wound care technologies should be utilized based on clinical findings, individualized care planning, and insurance. Continuous monitoring and reassessment in vascular status, offloading, compliance, and medical management are imperative in achieving diabetic foot ulcer healing. In this regard, nurses as members of the diabetic care team play a significant role in health care, public education, health system management, patient care and improving the quality of life, but must also attend in special training to use the latest instructions of diabetic foot care in order to provide effective management to facilitate, promote diabetic patient health, reduce sores and amputations. To prevent diabetic foot ulcer is multidisciplinary approach that have reduced the amputation rate, prevent complications, save cost and improve the standard of treatment by the team.

In our country, despite the increased number of diabetic patients, the training of specialist nurses such as diabetes or diabetic foot special nurses has not been considered. Maybe developing short term training courses for nurses, with the use of diabetic foot clinical guidelines and algorithms in clinics and hospitals will encourage nurses to enrol.

10.0 REFERENCES

1. World Health Organization (2015) Diabetes. Available at http://www.who.int, access on 6/3/2015.
2. Lavery LA, Ashry HR, van Houtum W, Pugh JA, Harkless LB, Basu S. Variation in the incidence and proportion of diabetes-related amputation in minorities, Diabetic Care 1996:48-52.
3. Van Netten, J. J.., Prince, P. E Lavery, L.A., Monteiro-Soares, M., Rasmussen, A. Jubiz, Y., Bus, S. A: Inter-

national Working Group on the Diabetic Foot Prevention of foot ulcers in the at-risk patient with diabetes: a systematic review. Diabetic Metabolism Research andReviews. 2016; 32 Suppl 1:84-98. Doi: 10.1002/dmrr.2701.

4. Sarwa N, Gao P, Seshasal SR, Gobin R, Kaptoge S, Di Angelantonio et al. Lancet. 2010; 26;375:2215-2222. Diabetic Mellitus, fasting blood glucose concentration, and risk of vascular diseases: a collaborative meta-analysis of 102 prospective studies. Emerging Risk Factors Collaboration.

5. Abbott CA, Carrington AL, Ashe H, Bath S, Every LC, Griffiths J, et al. The Notion foot care study: Incidence of and risk factors for, new diabetic foot ulceration based cohort. Diabetiv Med 2002;19:377-84.

6. Kruse I, Endelman S. Evaluation and treatment of diabetic ulceration 2006,24:91-3

7. Gibbons WG. Lower extremity bypass in patient with diabetic foot ulcers. Surg Clin Am 2003;83:659-669.

8. Singh N, Armstrong DG, Lipsky BA. Preventing foot ulcers in patients with diabetes LAMA 2005;293:217-228.

9. Mark AK, Warren SJ. Update of treatment of diabetic foot infections. Clin Podiatr Med Surg 2007;24:383-396.

10. James WB. Classification of foot lesions in Diabetic patients. Levin and O'Neals The Diabetic Foot. 2008;9:221-226.

11. Pecoraro RE, Reiber GE, Burgess EM. Pathways to diabetic limb amputation. Basis for prevention. Diabetic Care 1990;13:513-521.

12. Review The role of surgical debridement in healing of diabetic foot ulcers.

13. *Gordon KA, Lebrun EA, Tomic-Canic M, Kirsner RS. Skinmed. 2012 Jan-Feb; 10(1):24-6.*